TOP 25 NA
MEDICINE TO
REPAIR YOUR
LEAKY GUT

Eliminate Bloating, Indigestion
And Autoimmunity

By

Jocelyn Jones

TABLE OF CONTENTS

Introduction

A few years ago, I worked in a center that helped rehabilitate adults with various disorders and diseases. As someone who was passionate about health and wellness, I was always looking for new ways to help my clients heal and thrive.

It was during this time that I started to learn about leaky gut syndrome and its impact on overall health. I was shocked to discover that many people were suffering from this condition without even knowing it. I saw first-hand how leaky gut could lead to a range of health problems, from chronic inflammation to autoimmune disorders.

As I delved deeper into the research, I became more and more convinced that there had to be a better way to address leaky gut. While there were certainly medical interventions that could help, I felt that a more natural approach was needed.

That's when I started to compile the information that would eventually become my book, *"TOP 25 NATURAL MEDICINE TO REPAIR YOUR LEAKY GUT:* Eliminate Bloating, Indigestion, And Autoimmunity".

Drawing on my years of experience in the field, as well as the latest research on gut health, I put together a comprehensive guide to repairing leaky gut using natural remedies.

The book covers everything from the causes and symptoms of leaky gut to the best foods and supplements for healing. I also share personal stories from clients who have successfully overcome leaky gut using the methods outlined in the book.

Since publishing the book, I have received countless messages from readers who have been able to banish bloating, indigestion, and other gut issues using the natural remedies I recommend. It has been incredibly rewarding to see how the information in the book has helped people take control of their health and live their best lives.

As someone who has dedicated my career to helping others achieve optimal health and wellness, I am thrilled to be able to offer this resource to those struggling with leaky gut. I hope that it will serve as a valuable tool on your own journey to better health.

In this book, I share my knowledge and expertise on the subject of leaky gut syndrome and provide a comprehensive guide to repairing it using natural remedies.

Leaky gut is a condition that occurs when the lining of the small intestine becomes permeable, allowing harmful toxins, bacteria, and undigested food particles to leak into the bloodstream. This can lead to a range of health problems, including chronic inflammation, autoimmune disorders, and digestive issues such as bloating and indigestion.

While there are certainly medical interventions that can help with leaky gut, I believe that a more natural approach is often the best course of action. That's why I have compiled a list of the top 25 natural remedies that can help repair leaky gut and banish the associated symptoms.

Throughout this book, I will provide a detailed overview of leaky gut, including its causes, symptoms, and potential complications. I will also explain how the natural remedies included in this book can help heal and repair the gut lining, reduce inflammation, and restore optimal digestive function.

In addition to outlining the best natural remedies for leaky gut, I will also share tips on how to make lifestyle changes that can support gut health, including dietary changes and stress-reduction techniques. I will also provide advice on how to choose the best supplements and probiotics to support gut health.

This book is based on the latest research on leaky gut syndrome, as well as my years of experience working with clients who have struggled with this condition. It is my hope that the information and strategies outlined in this book will empower you to take control of your gut health and improve your overall well-being.

Thank you for choosing *"TOP 25 NATURAL MEDICINE TO REPAIR YOUR LEAKY GUT*: Banish Bloating, Indigestion, And Autoimmunity". Let's begin the journey to better gut health together.

What Is Leaky Gut?

Leaky gut, also known as increased intestinal permeability, is a condition where the lining of the small intestine becomes more porous than usual. Normally, the cells of the intestinal lining are tightly packed together, forming a barrier that prevents harmful substances from passing through into the bloodstream. However, when the intestinal lining becomes damaged or weakened, the spaces between the cells can widen, allowing substances such as toxins, undigested food particles, and bacteria to leak into the bloodstream.

The leaky gut phenomenon is not a new concept and has been known for decades in the medical community, but it has only recently gained more attention due to the rise of alternative medicine practices and the increasing evidence linking it to various health conditions.

There is no single cause of leaky gut, and it can be brought on by a variety of factors, including *chronic stress, poor diet, use of certain medications (such as nonsteroidal anti-inflammatory drugs), infections, and even aging.* Additionally, some medical conditions such as Crohn's disease, celiac disease, and irritable bowel syndrome have been associated with leaky gut.

When harmful substances leak into the bloodstream, they can trigger an immune response, causing inflammation in various parts of the body. This chronic inflammation can lead to a variety of health problems, including autoimmune disorders, allergies, skin conditions, and even mental health issues.

The symptoms of leaky gut can vary widely from person to person and can include bloating, gas, cramps, diarrhea or constipation, fatigue, headaches, joint pain, and skin rashes.

However, because these symptoms are nonspecific, leaky gut can be challenging to diagnose.

Fortunately, there are steps you can take to repair your gut lining and reduce the symptoms associated with leaky gut. This can include making dietary changes such as eliminating trigger foods, taking probiotics and other supplements, reducing stress levels, and getting enough sleep.

Overall, while there is still much to learn about leaky gut, research has shown that it is a real phenomenon that can have significant impacts on overall health. By understanding what leaky gut is and taking steps to address it, you can improve your gut health and potentially reduce your risk of associated health conditions.

How Does Leaky Gut Develop?

Leaky gut, also known as increased intestinal permeability, develops when the lining of the small intestine becomes more porous than usual. The intestinal lining is a vital barrier that separates the contents of the intestine from the bloodstream. It allows nutrients and other essential substances to pass through the lining and enter the bloodstream while preventing harmful substances such as toxins and bacteria from entering the bloodstream.

The lining of the small intestine is made up of a single layer of cells called enterocytes that are tightly packed together, forming a barrier known as the epithelial barrier. The enterocytes are connected to each other by tight junctions, which are protein structures that prevent substances from passing between the cells.

However, when the epithelial barrier is compromised, the tight junctions between the enterocytes become loose, and the spaces between the cells widen, allowing harmful substances to pass through the intestinal lining and enter the bloodstream. This condition is referred to as leaky gut.

Several factors can contribute to the development of leaky gut. Some of these factors include:

Poor Diet: A diet high in processed foods, sugar, and unhealthy fats can damage the intestinal lining and weaken the tight junctions between the enterocytes, leading to leaky gut.

Chronic Stress: Prolonged stress can disrupt the normal functioning of the gut, leading to inflammation and damage to the intestinal lining.

Use of Certain Medications: Certain medications, such as nonsteroidal anti-inflammatory drugs (NSAIDs), antibiotics, and chemotherapy drugs, can damage the intestinal lining and lead to leaky gut.

Infections: Certain infections, such as bacterial infections and parasitic infections, can damage the intestinal lining and lead to leaky gut.

Aging: As we age, the tight junctions between the enterocytes can become weaker, leading to leaky gut.

Medical Conditions: Certain medical conditions, such as Crohn's disease, celiac disease, and irritable bowel syndrome, have been associated with leaky gut.

When harmful substances pass through the intestinal lining and enter the bloodstream, they can trigger an immune response, leading to inflammation in various parts of the body. This chronic inflammation can lead to a variety of health problems, including autoimmune disorders, allergies, skin conditions, and even mental health issues.

Overall, while there is still much to learn about leaky gut, research has shown that it is a real phenomenon that can have significant impacts on overall health. By understanding the factors that can contribute to the development of leaky gut, you can take steps to protect your gut health and potentially reduce your risk of associated health conditions.

The Importance Of Gut Health

Gut health is a crucial aspect of overall health and wellbeing, as the gut plays a vital role in the body's digestive, immune, and metabolic functions. The gastrointestinal (GI) tract is a complex system that comprises various organs, including the stomach, small intestine, large intestine, and colon, as well as the liver, pancreas, and gallbladder. These organs work together to digest food, absorb nutrients, and eliminate waste products.

The importance of gut health can be seen in the many roles that the gut plays in the body:

Digestion: The gut is responsible for breaking down food into its component parts, including carbohydrates, proteins, and fats, and converting them into usable forms that the body can absorb.

Nutrient absorption: The gut absorbs nutrients from the food we eat, including vitamins, minerals, and other essential nutrients.

Immune function: The gut is home to trillions of bacteria, fungi, and other microorganisms that make up the gut microbiome. These microorganisms play a vital role in regulating the immune system and protecting against harmful pathogens.

Metabolism: The gut microbiome also plays a role in regulating metabolism and energy balance, which can impact overall health and weight management.

Hormone production: The gut produces hormones that regulate various bodily functions, including appetite and digestion.

Mood regulation: The gut-brain axis is a communication system between the gut and the brain, which allows for the regulation of mood and emotional well-being.

When the gut is functioning optimally, it can help promote overall health and wellbeing. However, when the gut is compromised, it can lead to a variety of health issues, including gastrointestinal disorders such as irritable bowel syndrome (IBS), inflammatory bowel disease (IBD), and gastroesophageal reflux disease (GERD). Poor gut health has also been linked to a range of other health problems, including autoimmune disorders, allergies, skin conditions, and even mental health issues such as anxiety and depression.

Therefore, it is important to take steps to maintain good gut health, such as consuming a healthy, balanced diet that is rich in fiber and probiotic-rich foods, staying hydrated, managing stress, and getting enough sleep. In addition, taking care of your gut microbiome by avoiding unnecessary antibiotics and using prebiotics and probiotics supplements can also support gut health. Overall, prioritizing gut health can help support overall health and wellbeing.

The Role of Natural Medicine in Gut Health

The role of natural medicine in gut health has become increasingly popular as people seek alternatives to traditional pharmaceuticals and medical interventions. Natural medicine refers to the use of natural remedies and therapies to promote health and prevent disease. The use of natural medicine for gut health can include dietary changes, nutritional supplements, herbal remedies, and other complementary therapies.

Dietary changes are an essential part of natural medicine for gut health. The food we eat has a significant impact on the health of our gut microbiome, which can affect our overall health. Eating a diet that is rich in fiber, whole foods, and plant-based sources of protein can help promote a healthy gut microbiome. Fermented foods, such as sauerkraut, kimchi, and kefir, can also be beneficial for gut health, as they contain beneficial bacteria that can help support the gut microbiome.

Nutritional supplements are another component of natural medicine for gut health. Probiotics, which are beneficial bacteria that help support the gut microbiome, can be taken in supplement form to help improve gut health. Prebiotics, which are foods that support the growth of beneficial bacteria in the gut, can also be taken in supplement form.

Herbal remedies can also be used to support gut health. Certain herbs, such as *ginger, chamomile, and peppermint,* have been used traditionally to soothe digestive discomfort and promote overall digestive health. Other herbs, such as *licorice root and slippery elm*, can be used to soothe the lining of the gut and reduce inflammation.

Other complementary therapies that can be used in natural medicine for gut health include acupuncture, massage therapy, and meditation. These therapies can help reduce stress, which can have a negative impact on gut health, and promote relaxation, which can help support digestive function.

Overall, the role of natural medicine in gut health is to support the body's natural healing mechanisms and promote optimal digestive function. By making dietary changes, taking nutritional supplements, using herbal remedies, and other complementary therapies, individuals can support their gut health and promote overall health and wellbeing. However, it is important to note that natural medicine should not replace traditional medical care and advice, and individuals should always consult with a healthcare professional before making any significant changes to their diet or healthcare routine.

CHAPTER 1

Understanding Leaky Gut Syndrome

Leaky gut syndrome is a condition in which the lining of the gut becomes more permeable than normal, allowing toxins, bacteria, and other harmful substances to pass through the gut lining and into the bloodstream. This can lead to inflammation, food sensitivities, and other health issues.

The lining of the gut is designed to be selective, allowing nutrients to pass through while keeping harmful substances out. However, when the gut becomes more permeable, this selective function is compromised. The result is that larger molecules, such as undigested food particles, toxins, and bacteria, can enter the bloodstream.

Leaky gut syndrome can be caused by a variety of reasons. These include *a poor diet that is high in processed foods and sugar, chronic stress, the use of certain medications such as antibiotics and nonsteroidal anti-inflammatory drugs (NSAIDs), and exposure to environmental toxins.*

When harmful substances enter the bloodstream through the gut lining, the body's immune system responds by triggering an inflammatory response. This can lead to a wide range of symptoms, including digestive issues such as bloating, gas, and diarrhea, as well as skin issues, fatigue, joint pain, and brain fog.

The diagnosis of leaky gut syndrome can be difficult, as it is not currently recognized as a medical condition by many healthcare professionals. However, there are a number of tests that can be used to assess gut health, including stool tests, blood tests, and breath tests.

The treatment of leaky gut syndrome typically involves a multifaceted approach. This may include dietary changes to eliminate foods that are known to contribute to gut inflammation, such as processed foods, sugar, and gluten. It may also involve the use of nutritional supplements to support gut healing, such as probiotics, digestive enzymes, and glutamine.

In addition to dietary and supplement interventions, other lifestyle factors may also be addressed in the treatment of leaky gut syndrome. This may include stress management techniques such as meditation and yoga, as well as regular exercise and sufficient sleep.

Overall, understanding leaky gut syndrome is an important step in addressing gut health and promoting overall wellbeing. By identifying the factors that contribute to the development of leaky gut syndrome and implementing a multifaceted approach to treatment, individuals can support their gut health and reduce the risk of associated health issues.

The link between leaky gut and bloating, indigestion, and autoimmune issues.

Leaky gut syndrome is a condition that occurs when the intestinal lining becomes more permeable, allowing toxins, undigested food particles, and harmful bacteria to leak out of the gut and into the bloodstream. This can lead to a host of health problems, including bloating, indigestion, and autoimmune issues.

Bloating is a common symptom of leaky gut syndrome. When the gut lining becomes compromised, it can lead to inflammation, which can cause gas and bloating. Additionally, the presence of undigested food particles and toxins in the bloodstream can further exacerbate these symptoms.

Indigestion is another common symptom of leaky gut syndrome. When the gut lining is compromised, it can lead to poor nutrient absorption and digestive issues. This can cause discomfort, pain, and a range of other symptoms, including heartburn, nausea, and vomiting.

Autoimmune issues are also linked to leaky gut syndrome. When the gut lining becomes more permeable, it can lead to the release of toxins and undigested food particles into the bloodstream. This can trigger an immune response, leading to the development of autoimmune conditions such as rheumatoid arthritis, lupus, and celiac disease.

It is important to note that not all cases of bloating, indigestion, and autoimmune issues are caused by leaky gut syndrome. However, research suggests that improving gut health through the use of natural medicine can be beneficial in managing these symptoms, and potentially even reversing the underlying condition.

The Importance Of Natural Medicine In Healing Leaky Gut

Leaky gut syndrome can have a significant impact on overall health, leading to a range of symptoms and contributing to the development of chronic conditions. While conventional medicine can be helpful in managing some of these symptoms, natural medicine approaches can play an important role in healing leaky gut and restoring gut health.

One of the primary benefits of natural medicine in the treatment of leaky gut is its focus on addressing the root causes of the condition. This may involve a holistic approach that considers not only the physical symptoms of leaky gut, but also factors such as stress, diet, and lifestyle habits that can contribute to the condition.

Natural medicine approaches to leaky gut may include dietary changes, such as avoiding trigger foods that can exacerbate symptoms, and increasing intake of nutrient-dense foods that promote gut health. Supplements and herbs may also be used to support gut healing and reduce inflammation, such as probiotics, digestive enzymes, and anti-inflammatory herbs like turmeric and ginger.

Other natural medicine approaches to healing leaky gut may include stress management techniques like meditation and yoga, as stress can contribute to gut inflammation and compromise gut health. Lifestyle changes, such as getting adequate sleep and exercise, can also play a role in supporting gut health and reducing symptoms of leaky gut syndrome.

Natural medicine approaches can also be effective in addressing co-occurring conditions that may contribute to leaky gut, such as autoimmune conditions or chronic infections. By addressing these underlying conditions, natural medicine approaches can help to restore gut health and promote overall well-being.

Overall, the importance of natural medicine in healing leaky gut lies in its ability to take a holistic, root-cause approach to treatment, supporting the body's natural healing processes and promoting optimal gut health.

CHAPTER 2

The Basics of Healing Leaky Gut

Healing leaky gut is a multi-faceted process that involves addressing various factors that contribute to gut inflammation and compromised gut health. Here are some of the basic principles of healing leaky gut:

Remove Triggers: The first step in healing leaky gut is to identify and remove any triggers that may be contributing to gut inflammation. This may include eliminating foods that are causing an immune response, such as gluten, dairy, and processed foods, as well as addressing any underlying infections or other conditions that may be contributing to gut inflammation.

Repair the Gut Lining: Once triggers have been removed, the focus shifts to repairing the damaged gut lining. This may involve incorporating nutrients that are essential for gut healing, such as collagen, glutamine, and zinc, as well as supplementing with probiotics and digestive enzymes to support gut flora and aid digestion.

Reduce Inflammation: Inflammation is a key contributor to leaky gut syndrome, so reducing inflammation is an important part of the healing process. This may involve incorporating anti-inflammatory foods and herbs into the diet, such as turmeric, ginger, and omega-3 fatty acids, as well as addressing any underlying conditions that may be contributing to inflammation, such as autoimmune disorders or chronic infections.

Restore Gut Flora: Gut bacteria play a crucial role in gut health, so restoring the balance of gut flora is essential in healing leaky gut. This may involve supplementing with probiotics and prebiotics, as well as incorporating fermented foods like sauerkraut, kimchi, and kefir into the diet.

Support Digestion: Proper digestion is key in preventing gut inflammation and leaky gut syndrome. Supporting digestion may involve incorporating digestive aids like digestive enzymes and herbs like ginger and peppermint, as well as reducing stress and avoiding overeating.

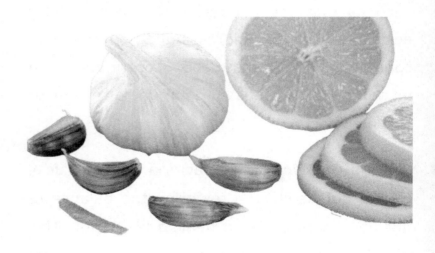

Understanding The Digestive System And How It Works

The digestive system is an essential part of the human body responsible for breaking down food into nutrients that can be absorbed and used by the body. It is composed of a series of organs that work together to ensure efficient digestion and absorption of nutrients.

The process of digestion begins in the mouth, where the teeth and tongue break down food into smaller pieces and mix it with saliva. This saliva contains enzymes that start the process of breaking down carbohydrates.

Once the food is swallowed, it enters the esophagus and moves down to the stomach. The stomach secretes acid and enzymes that break down proteins and fats, while also continuing the digestion of carbohydrates.

After leaving the stomach, the partially digested food enters the small intestine, where most of the nutrients are absorbed. The small intestine is lined with villi and microvilli, which increase the surface area and allow for efficient absorption of nutrients.

The large intestine, also known as the colon, is responsible for absorbing water and electrolytes, while also producing and storing feces until elimination.

Throughout this process, the digestive system works in concert with the nervous and endocrine systems to regulate digestion and ensure proper nutrient absorption.

Understanding how the digestive system works is crucial for maintaining gut health and preventing digestive disorders such as leaky gut syndrome. By supporting the digestive system with proper nutrition and lifestyle choices, we can optimize its function and promote overall health and well-being.

The Causes Of Leaky Gut Syndrome

Leaky gut syndrome is a condition where the lining of the small intestine becomes damaged, allowing undigested food particles, toxins, and other harmful substances to leak into the bloodstream. This can cause a wide range of health issues, including autoimmune disorders, allergies, and digestive problems.

Leaky gut syndrome has a number of potential causes, such as:

Poor diet: A diet high in processed foods, sugar, and refined carbohydrates can lead to inflammation in the gut and damage to the intestinal lining.

Chronic stress: Prolonged stress can disrupt the balance of beneficial bacteria in the gut and compromise the intestinal lining.

Overuse of antibiotics: Antibiotics can disrupt the balance of gut bacteria, leading to an overgrowth of harmful bacteria and damage to the intestinal lining.

Environmental toxins: Exposure to environmental toxins such as pesticides, heavy metals, and pollution can damage the gut lining and lead to leaky gut syndrome.

Chronic inflammation: Conditions such as inflammatory bowel disease (IBD) and celiac disease can cause chronic inflammation in the gut, which can lead to damage to the intestinal lining.

Aging: As we age, the integrity of the intestinal lining can deteriorate, leading to leaky gut syndrome.

It's important to note that leaky gut syndrome is a complex condition with multiple contributing factors. Identifying the root causes and addressing them through diet, lifestyle changes, and natural medicine can help to heal the gut lining and promote overall health and wellness.

Symptoms Of Leaky Gut

Leaky gut syndrome is a condition that can have a wide range of symptoms, which can make it difficult to diagnose. However, there are some common symptoms that are associated with this condition. These include:

Digestive issues: Digestive issues are one of the most common symptoms of leaky gut syndrome. This can include bloating, gas, diarrhea, constipation, and stomach pain.

Food intolerances: People with leaky gut syndrome may develop food intolerances or sensitivities, particularly to foods that are high in FODMAPs (fermentable oligo-, di-, and monosaccharides and polyols) or gluten.

Skin Issues: Skin issues, such as eczema, psoriasis, and acne, are often linked to leaky gut syndrome.

Fatigue: Chronic fatigue or exhaustion is a common symptom of leaky gut syndrome.

Joint Pain: Joint pain or stiffness is another common symptom of leaky gut syndrome, particularly in the hips, knees, and lower back.

Brain fog: Brain fog or difficulty concentrating is another common symptom of leaky gut syndrome.

Autoimmune Conditions: Leaky gut syndrome has been linked to autoimmune conditions, such as rheumatoid arthritis, multiple sclerosis, and Hashimoto's thyroiditis.

It's important to note that these symptoms can also be caused by other conditions, so it's important to work with a healthcare professional to determine if leaky gut syndrome is the cause.

The Impact Of Leaky Gut On Health

Leaky gut syndrome is a condition that can have a significant impact on overall health. The digestive system plays a crucial role in keeping the body healthy by absorbing nutrients, eliminating waste, and supporting the immune system. When the gut becomes permeable and allows toxins, undigested food particles, and bacteria to enter the bloodstream, it can cause inflammation and trigger an immune response.

The chronic inflammation that results from a leaky gut can contribute to a range of health problems. It can disrupt the balance of gut bacteria, known as the gut microbiome, and cause an overgrowth of harmful bacteria. This imbalance can lead to a variety of digestive problems, including bloating, gas, and diarrhea. Over time, chronic inflammation can also lead to more serious conditions, including autoimmune diseases, such as rheumatoid arthritis, multiple sclerosis, and type 1 diabetes.

Leaky gut syndrome has also been linked to mental health issues, including anxiety and depression. Chronic inflammation can affect the production of neurotransmitters in the brain, leading to imbalances that can cause mood disorders.

In addition to affecting the gut and mental health, leaky gut syndrome can also impact other areas of the body. Chronic inflammation can contribute to skin problems, such as eczema and psoriasis. It can also contribute to allergies and food sensitivities, as the immune system becomes hypersensitive to certain substances.

The impact of leaky gut on health can be significant and far-reaching. It is essential to address this condition through natural medicine and lifestyle changes to promote gut health and prevent further damage to the body.

How To Test For Leaky Gut

Leaky gut syndrome is a condition that affects the lining of the intestines, allowing harmful substances to leak into the bloodstream. Testing for leaky gut involves a variety of methods, and while none of them are foolproof, they can provide useful information to help diagnose and treat the condition.

One common method for testing for leaky gut is the lactulose/mannitol test. In this test, the patient drinks a solution containing lactulose and mannitol, two types of sugars that the body does not absorb. The patient then collects a urine sample over the next six hours, which is tested for the levels of lactulose and mannitol. If the levels of lactulose are higher than the levels of mannitol, it suggests that the patient has increased intestinal permeability and may have leaky gut syndrome.

Another method for testing for leaky gut is the zonulin test. A protein called zonulin controls the tight junctions that separate intestinal cells. Elevated levels of zonulin can indicate increased intestinal permeability and leaky gut syndrome.

Doctors may also order blood tests to look for antibodies to certain proteins found in the gut. These antibodies can indicate that the body is reacting to substances that have leaked through the gut lining.

In addition to these tests, doctors may also use other methods to diagnose leaky gut syndrome, such as stool analysis or endoscopy.

It is important to note that while these tests can provide useful information, they are not always conclusive. There is still much research to be done on leaky gut syndrome and its diagnosis and treatment, and doctors may use a combination of methods to arrive at a diagnosis.

The Role Of Diet And Lifestyle In Healing Leaky Gut

The role of diet and lifestyle cannot be overstated when it comes to healing leaky gut. The food we eat and the habits we engage in can significantly affect the health of our gut. Here are some notes on the importance of diet and lifestyle in healing leaky gut:

Elimination Diet: One of the first steps in healing leaky gut is to identify and eliminate the foods that are causing inflammation and damage to the gut lining. This can be done through an elimination diet, where you remove common allergens and inflammatory foods like gluten, dairy, soy, corn, and processed foods from your diet for a period of time.

Nutrient-Dense Foods: Eating a nutrient-dense diet that is rich in vitamins, minerals, and antioxidants can help to repair the gut lining and support the growth of beneficial bacteria in the gut. Include plenty of fresh vegetables and fruits, lean proteins, healthy fats, and probiotic-rich foods like fermented vegetables, kefir, and yogurt.

Hydration: Adequate hydration is essential for maintaining the health of the gut. Avoid sugary drinks and alcohol, and make an effort to consume at least 8 to 10 glasses of water each day.

Stress Management: Chronic stress can have a negative impact on the gut, causing inflammation and damage to the gut lining. Incorporating stress-management techniques like meditation, yoga, and deep breathing can help to reduce stress and support gut health.

Sleep: Getting adequate sleep is important for the health of the gut. Aim for 7-8 hours of sleep per night, and establish a regular sleep routine.

Exercise: Regular exercise can help to improve gut health by reducing inflammation, promoting regular bowel movements, and increasing the diversity of gut bacteria. An ideal amount of daily moderate exercise is 30 minutes.

Probiotics And Prebiotics: Probiotics are beneficial bacteria that can help to improve the balance of gut bacteria and support the health of the gut. Prebiotics are foods that feed the beneficial bacteria in the gut. Incorporating probiotic-rich foods like fermented vegetables, kefir, and yogurt, as well as prebiotic-rich foods like onions, garlic, and asparagus, can help to support gut health.

In summary, healing leaky gut requires a comprehensive approach that includes dietary and lifestyle changes. Eliminating inflammatory foods, eating a nutrient-dense diet, staying hydrated, managing stress, getting adequate sleep, exercising regularly, and incorporating probiotics and prebiotics into your diet can all help to support the health of the gut and promote healing.

CHAPTER 3:

The Top 6 Natural Medicines For Repairing Leaky Gut

PROBIOTICS

Probiotics are live microorganisms that are beneficial for human health, especially the digestive system. These microorganisms can be found naturally in certain fermented foods such as yogurt, kefir, kimchi, sauerkraut, and miso, or they can be taken as dietary supplements.

Probiotics work by restoring and balancing the gut microbiome, which is the community of microorganisms that live in the digestive tract. A healthy gut microbiome plays a crucial role in overall health by helping to digest food, synthesizing vitamins, regulating the immune system, and even influencing mood.

Research has shown that probiotics can help improve digestive health by reducing symptoms such as bloating, gas, constipation, and diarrhea. Probiotics may also have benefits for other conditions such as allergies, eczema, and respiratory infections.

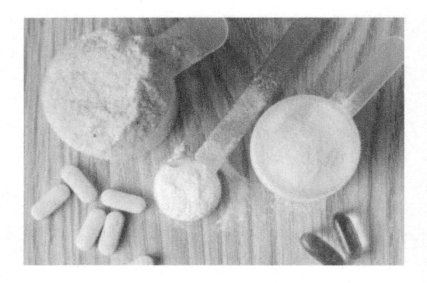

Not all probiotics are made equal, it is crucial to remember this. Different strains of bacteria have different effects on the body, so it is important to choose a probiotic supplement that is specifically designed for the condition being treated. Additionally, the dosage and frequency of probiotic use may vary depending on the individual's needs and the severity of the condition.

While probiotics are generally considered safe, individuals with compromised immune systems or serious medical conditions should consult with a healthcare professional before taking them.

DIGESTIVE ENZYMES

Digestive enzymes are substances that the body produces naturally to help break down food and facilitate the absorption of nutrients. They are produced by various organs in the digestive system, including the pancreas, stomach, and small intestine.

The three main types of digestive enzymes are:

Proteases: These enzymes break down proteins into their individual amino acids.

Lipases: These enzymes break down fats into their component fatty acids and glycerol.

Amylases: These enzymes, known as amylases, convert carbs into simple sugars.

When the digestive system is functioning properly, the body produces enough digestive enzymes to break down the food we eat. However, when there is a deficiency of digestive enzymes, food may not be fully digested, leading to discomfort and other digestive issues.

There are many factors that can contribute to a deficiency of digestive enzymes, *including aging, poor diet, and certain medical conditions.*

To address this deficiency, digestive enzyme supplements can be taken to help break down food and improve digestion.

Digestive enzymes can be beneficial for individuals with various digestive issues, including bloating, gas, constipation, and diarrhea. However, it is important to talk to a healthcare professional before starting any new supplements or making significant changes to your diet or lifestyle

L-GLUTAMINE

L-glutamine is an amino acid that plays a vital role in the body. The bloodstream contains the highest concentration of this amino acid, which is crucial for numerous cellular processes. L-glutamine is primarily used to promote gut health, as it is a building block for the cells lining the digestive tract. It is also essential for maintaining the integrity of the intestinal lining and can aid in repairing a leaky gut.

One of the key ways L-glutamine helps to heal leaky gut is by strengthening the tight junctions in the intestinal lining. These tight junctions are responsible for keeping harmful substances from passing through the gut wall and into the bloodstream. When the gut becomes leaky, these tight junctions become weak and allow toxins, undigested food particles, and other harmful substances to enter the bloodstream, leading to inflammation and other health issues.

L-glutamine can also help to reduce inflammation in the gut, which is a significant contributing factor to leaky gut syndrome. Chronic inflammation can damage the gut lining, making it more permeable and leading to the development of leaky gut.

Additionally, L-glutamine has been shown to support the growth of beneficial bacteria in the gut. These beneficial bacteria play a crucial role in maintaining gut health and can help to reduce inflammation, boost immunity, and improve overall digestive function.

Supplementing with L-glutamine can help to improve gut health and repair a leaky gut. It is available in powder or capsule form, and it is generally considered safe when taken at recommended doses. However, it is always essential to consult with a healthcare provider before starting any new supplement regimen, especially if you have a medical condition or are taking medications.

LICORICE ROOT

Licorice root, also known as *Glycyrrhiza glabra*, has been used for centuries in traditional medicine to treat various ailments, including digestive issues. It contains numerous active compounds, including glycyrrhizin, which gives it a characteristic sweet taste, and flavonoids, such as *liquiritin* and *isoliquiritin*. Licorice root has been found to have anti-inflammatory, antioxidant, and antimicrobial properties, which makes it a potentially effective treatment for leaky gut syndrome.

One of the key benefits of licorice root is its ability to reduce inflammation in the gut. Chronic inflammation is a major contributor to the development of leaky gut syndrome, and licorice root has been shown to reduce inflammatory markers in the gut, such as TNF-alpha and IL-6. By reducing inflammation, licorice root can help to repair the intestinal lining and improve gut health.

Licorice root has also been found to have antioxidant properties, which can help to protect the gut from damage caused by free radicals. Free radicals are unstable molecules that can damage cells and tissues, and they are thought to contribute to the development of many chronic diseases, including leaky gut syndrome. By neutralizing free radicals, licorice root can help to protect the gut from damage and promote healing.

In addition to its anti-inflammatory and antioxidant properties, licorice root also has antimicrobial effects. It has been found to be effective against a variety of harmful bacteria, viruses, and fungi, including H. pylori, a bacteria that is associated with the development of ulcers and leaky gut syndrome. By reducing the presence of harmful microorganisms in the gut, licorice root can help to restore the balance of gut bacteria and improve overall gut health.

Overall, licorice root is a promising natural medicine for the treatment of leaky gut syndrome. Its anti-inflammatory, antioxidant, and antimicrobial properties make it a potentially effective treatment for reducing inflammation, protecting against damage, and promoting healing in the gut. However, as with all natural medicines, it is important to consult with a healthcare provider before using licorice root as a treatment for leaky gut syndrome.

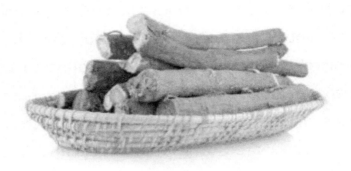

SLIPPERY ELM

Slippery elm is an herb that has been used for centuries by indigenous people to treat various ailments, including digestive issues. It comes from the inner bark of the slippery elm tree, and it has a high mucilage content, which makes it a natural demulcent. The mucilage in slippery elm helps to soothe and protect the lining of the digestive tract, making it an effective natural medicine for healing leaky gut.

Slippery elm is also rich in antioxidants, which help to protect the body from oxidative stress and inflammation. These antioxidants include vitamin C, beta-carotene, quercetin, and kaempferol, among others. Additionally, slippery elm contains anti-inflammatory compounds, such as tannins, which can help to reduce inflammation in the digestive tract and promote healing.

One of the key benefits of slippery elm for leaky gut is its ability to promote the growth of healthy gut bacteria. This is because the mucilage in slippery elm acts as a prebiotic, which feeds the beneficial bacteria in the gut. By supporting the growth of healthy gut bacteria, slippery elm can help to restore balance to the gut microbiome and improve overall gut health.

Slippery elm can be taken as a supplement in capsule or powder form, or it can be consumed as a tea. To make slippery elm tea, simply mix one teaspoon of powdered slippery elm bark with one cup of boiling water, and let it steep for 10-15 minutes before drinking. It is important to note that slippery elm may interact with certain medications, so it is always best to consult with a healthcare provider before taking any new supplements or herbs.

CAPRYLIC ACID

Caprylic acid is a medium-chain fatty acid found in coconut oil that provides many health benefits. It has strong anti-inflammatory properties that can promote good gut health and relieve symptoms of leaky gut caused by inflammation. In overweight and obese individuals, consuming caprylic acid can help remodel gut microbiota, improve lipid metabolism, prevent intestinal permeability, and reduce unhealthy fat storage.

Caprylic acid also has antibacterial properties that make it an effective natural remedy for people with leaky gut. Bad bacteria and inflammation can cause gut health issues, but caprylic acid can help combat them. It can also improve the intestinal barrier, especially in overweight and obese individuals who are trying to lose weight.

Consuming caprylic acid can be achieved by adding coconut oil to the diet or taking supplements. If you choose to ingest coconut oil, it's recommended to start with a small amount, such as one tablespoon. Caprylic acid supplements are also widely available in stores where supplements are sold.

Overall, caprylic acid is a powerful natural remedy for improving gut health, especially for those with leaky gut or who are overweight or obese. Adding it to your diet or taking

supplements can provide many health benefits
and improve overall wellness.

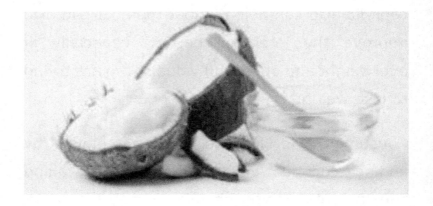

CHAPTER 4

The Top 5 Natural Medicines For Banishing Bloating

PEPPERMINT OIL AND THYME

Peppermint, a commonly known herb from the mint family, is known for its revitalizing aroma and extensive benefits. The essential oils found in peppermint leaves, including menthol, menthone, and limonene, give the plant its energizing aroma and cooling effect. It has various benefits that can positively impact your health, including its usefulness in aiding digestion, relaxing the digestive system, easing pain, and preventing gut spasms.

Peppermint has antioxidant and immune-boosting effects that enhance your overall well-being. Studies have shown that consumption of peppermint improves gastrointestinal scores and can be used as a natural remedy for digestive issues. Peppermint oil can relieve abdominal pain and aid the management of symptoms associated with irritable bowel syndrome (IBS), such as constipation, diarrhea, and bloating. It also has an anti-inflammatory effect, which helps in repairing leaky gut.

Peppermint can significantly reduce the severity of gut symptoms and make you feel calm. Thyme, another herb that can help in repairing leaky gut, strengthens intestinal integrity and increases the value of total antioxidant status. It also supports the growth of good bacteria in your gut, which is essential in maintaining gut health.

Both peppermint and thyme can be used in various ways, including using fresh or dried leaves to complement dishes or making tea. They can also be ingested in oil form in teas, smoothies, or other beverages. Incorporating these herbs into your diet can help improve your gut health and alleviate digestive issues.

However, peppermint oil is a popular natural medicine known for its ability to alleviate digestive issues, including bloating. It is derived from the peppermint plant, a hybrid of water mint and spearmint, and has a long history of use in traditional medicine for its antispasmodic and carminative properties.

Peppermint oil helps to relieve bloating by relaxing the muscles in the digestive tract, allowing for easier passage of gas and stool. It also has a cooling effect on the digestive system, which can help to soothe inflammation and irritation that can contribute to bloating.

Research has shown that peppermint oil can be effective in reducing symptoms of irritable bowel syndrome (IBS), a condition that often includes bloating as a symptom. One study found that a combination of peppermint oil and caraway oil significantly reduced bloating in patients with IBS compared to a placebo group.

Peppermint oil is available in various forms, including capsules, tablets, and liquid extracts. It is important to follow the recommended dosage instructions provided on the product label, as high doses can cause side effects such as nausea and heartburn.

Peppermint oil is generally considered safe for most people when used as directed. However, it should be used with caution in individuals with certain medical conditions, such as gastroesophageal reflux disease (GERD), as it can worsen symptoms in some cases. It is also not recommended for use in infants and young children.

Overall, peppermint oil is a natural medicine that can be a helpful addition to a comprehensive approach to managing bloating Before using any supplement, as with any other dietary addition, it is advised to see a healthcare professional, especially if you have any underlying medical concerns or are taking any drugs.

Tip: You can try adding fresh or dried peppermint and thyme leaves to your meals or drinking peppermint or thyme tea to enjoy their benefits. You can also use peppermint or thyme oil in your smoothies or other beverages.

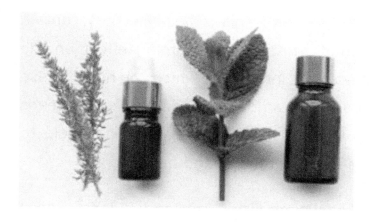

FENNEL SEEDS

Fennel seeds have been used for centuries for medicinal purposes, particularly for digestive issues. The seeds come from the fennel plant, which is native to the Mediterranean region but is now grown in many parts of the world.

One of the key benefits of fennel seeds is their ability to reduce bloating and gas in the digestive system. This is because they contain compounds that have a calming effect on the muscles in the intestines, which can help to ease spasms and cramps. In addition, fennel seeds have a mild diuretic effect, which can help to reduce water retention and bloating.

Fennel seeds are also rich in antioxidants, which can help to reduce inflammation in the body. This is important because chronic inflammation is thought to be a contributing factor to many health problems, including digestive issues.

Studies have shown that fennel seeds may be particularly effective for treating irritable bowel syndrome (IBS). In one study, patients with IBS who took fennel seed oil capsules experienced a significant reduction in symptoms such as bloating, abdominal pain, and flatulence.

Fennel seeds can be consumed in a variety of ways, such as chewing on the seeds directly or brewing them as a tea. Fennel seed tea is easy to make by steeping a teaspoon of seeds in hot water for several minutes.

Overall, fennel seeds are a safe and natural remedy for bloating and other digestive issues. They are easy to incorporate into your diet and can be a useful addition to other natural remedies for digestive health.

GINGER

Ginger has been used for centuries in traditional medicine to aid digestion and alleviate digestive discomfort. It contains several active compounds, including **gingerols** and **shogaols,** that have anti-inflammatory and antioxidant properties.

Here are some of the ways in which ginger can help with bloating:

Reduces inflammation: Ginger contains compounds that have anti-inflammatory properties, which can help reduce inflammation in the digestive tract. This, in turn, can help relieve bloating caused by inflammation.

Stimulates digestion: Ginger has been shown to stimulate the production of digestive juices and enzymes, which can help break down food more effectively and prevent bloating caused by indigestion.

Relieves gas: Ginger has carminative properties, which means it can help relieve gas and bloating by relaxing the muscles in the digestive tract.

Soothes nausea: Ginger has been shown to be effective at reducing nausea, which can be a common symptom of bloating.

There are several ways to incorporate ginger into your diet, such as adding it to *smoothies, teas, or using it in cooking*. Ginger supplements are also available in capsule form, but it is always best to consult with a healthcare professional before starting any new supplements.

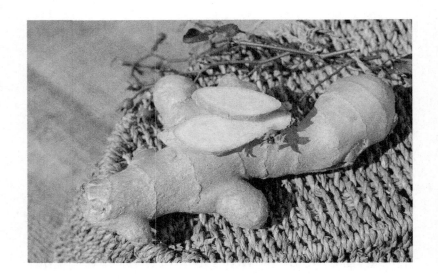

CHAMOMILE

Chamomile is an herb that has been used for centuries for its medicinal properties. It is commonly used to promote relaxation and reduce stress, but it also has many benefits for digestive health. Chamomile is derived from the daisy-like flowers of the chamomile plant, and it is typically consumed as a tea or taken in supplement form.

One of the primary benefits of chamomile is its ability to soothe the digestive tract. Chamomile contains compounds that can help to reduce inflammation and irritation in the digestive system. This can be particularly helpful for individuals who suffer from bloating and other digestive issues.

Chamomile has also been shown to have a calming effect on the body, which can help to reduce stress and anxiety. When the body is under stress, it can have a negative impact on digestive health, leading to issues like bloating and indigestion. By promoting relaxation, chamomile can help to alleviate these symptoms.

Another benefit of chamomile is its ability to reduce muscle spasms in the digestive tract. This can be helpful for individuals who suffer from conditions like irritable bowel syndrome (IBS), which is characterized by abdominal pain and cramping.

Overall, chamomile is a safe and natural remedy that can be used to promote digestive health and alleviate symptoms like bloating and indigestion. It can be consumed as a tea or taken in supplement form, and it is generally well-tolerated with few side effects. However, individuals with allergies to ragweed or other plants in the daisy family may need to exercise caution when using chamomile

CARAWAY SEEDS

Caraway seeds have been used for centuries as a natural remedy to aid digestion, relieve bloating and gas, and improve overall gut health. They are commonly used in traditional European cuisine and can be added to various dishes such as soups, stews, and bread.

Caraway seeds are rich in antioxidants, vitamins, and minerals such as *calcium, magnesium, and iron*. They also contain essential oils that have *antibacterial* and *antifungal* properties, which can help in preventing gut infections and promoting a healthy gut flora.

One of the main benefits of caraway seeds is their ability to stimulate the production of digestive enzymes and gastric juices in the stomach, which helps in breaking down food and easing digestion. They are also known to have a **carminative effect**, which means they help in reducing gas and bloating.

Studies have shown that caraway seeds can also help in *reducing inflammation in the gut*, which is a common factor in many digestive disorders such as **irritable bowel syndrome (IBS)** and **Crohn's disease**. They can also help in preventing the growth of harmful bacteria in the gut, while promoting the growth of beneficial bacteria.

Caraway seeds can be consumed in various ways, including adding them to **meals, brewing them as tea**, **or taking them in supplement** form. However, it is important to note that they may cause allergic reactions in some individuals, and should be avoided by pregnant women.

Caraway seeds are a natural and effective way to improve digestion, reduce bloating and gas, and promote gut health.

CHAPTER 5

The Top 5 Natural Medicines for Relieving Indigestion:

APPLE CIDER VINEGAR

Apple cider vinegar (ACV) is a popular natural remedy that has been used for centuries to alleviate various health issues, including indigestion. It is made by fermenting crushed apples with yeast and bacteria to convert the natural sugars into acetic acid. ACV is known for its antibacterial and anti-inflammatory properties, which can help improve digestion and reduce inflammation in the gut.

Here are some ways ACV can help relieve indigestion:

Stomach Acid: ACV contains acetic acid, which can help stimulate the production of stomach acid. This can be helpful for individuals who have low stomach acid, which can cause indigestion.

Digestive Enzymes: ACV contains enzymes that can aid in digestion by breaking down food molecules. This may lessen gas and bloating.

Anti-inflammatory: ACV has anti-inflammatory properties that can help reduce inflammation in the gut, which is a common cause of indigestion.

Probiotics: ACV contains probiotics, which are beneficial bacteria that can help improve gut health and aid in digestion.

Here are some ways to use ACV to relieve indigestion:

Drink ACV before meals: Mix 1-2 tablespoons of ACV with water and drink before meals to stimulate the production of stomach acid and aid in digestion.

Use ACV in dressings and marinades: Add ACV to salad dressings and marinades to improve digestion and reduce inflammation.

Take ACV capsules: ACV capsules are available at health food stores and can be taken as a supplement to aid in digestion.

Use ACV as a natural antacid: Mix 1 tablespoon of ACV with water and drink to alleviate symptoms of indigestion, such as heartburn.

Overall, ACV is a natural and effective way to relieve indigestion. However, it is important to note that ACV is acidic and should be consumed in moderation. Excessive consumption of ACV can damage tooth enamel and irritate the digestive tract. It is recommended to dilute ACV with water and consume in moderation.

ALOE VERA

Aloe vera is a succulent plant with thick and fleshy leaves that contain a clear gel. This plant has been used for centuries as a natural remedy for a variety of health conditions. One of its well-known uses is for relieving indigestion.

Aloe vera contains compounds called polysaccharides that help soothe and heal the lining of the digestive tract. It also has anti-inflammatory properties that can reduce inflammation in the gut, which is often the cause of indigestion.

In addition to these benefits, aloe vera has a mild laxative effect that can help promote regular bowel movements and reduce constipation, which can also contribute to indigestion. The plant also has antibacterial and antifungal properties that can help kill off harmful bacteria in the gut that may be causing indigestion

One of the most convenient ways to use aloe vera for indigestion is to drink aloe vera juice. This juice is widely available at health food stores and online. It is important to note that not all aloe vera juice products are created equal, and some may contain added sugars or other ingredients that can be irritating to the digestive system. It is best to look for a high-quality, pure aloe vera juice product that is free from additives.

Another way to use aloe vera for indigestion is to consume the gel directly from the plant. To do this, simply cut open a leaf of the aloe vera plant and scoop out the gel with a spoon. This can be added to smoothies or other beverages, or consumed on its own.

Overall, aloe vera is a safe and effective natural remedy for relieving indigestion. It is important to consult with a healthcare provider before using aloe vera or any other natural remedy,

particularly if you are pregnant or have any
medical conditions.

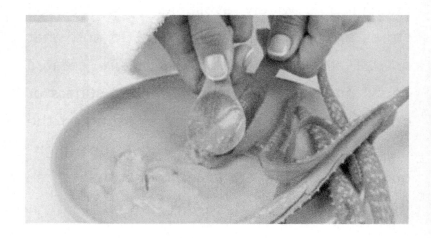

MARSHMALLOW ROOT

Marshmallow root is an herb commonly used in traditional medicine to treat a range of ailments, including digestive issues. It is especially effective in alleviating symptoms of indigestion, heartburn, and acid reflux. Marshmallow root is rich in mucilage, a gel-like substance that can soothe and protect the lining of the digestive tract.

One of the primary benefits of marshmallow root is its ability to reduce inflammation in the digestive system. Inflammation can damage the sensitive lining of the digestive tract, causing discomfort and pain. The mucilage in marshmallow root can help to reduce inflammation, thus relieving symptoms of indigestion and other digestive issues.

Marshmallow root is also beneficial for increasing the production of mucous in the stomach. This can help to protect the stomach lining from the corrosive effects of stomach acid, reducing the risk of developing stomach ulcers.

Furthermore, marshmallow root can help to regulate bowel movements and promote healthy digestion. It has a mild laxative effect that can help to relieve constipation and improve overall gut health.

Marshmallow root can be consumed as a tea, capsule, or extract. It is generally considered safe and well-tolerated, although some people may experience mild side effects such as bloating or diarrhea. As with any natural supplement, it is important to consult with a healthcare provider before using marshmallow root to treat digestive issues.

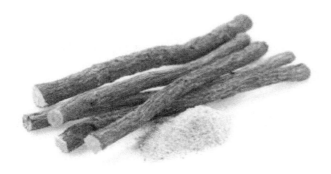

DANDELION ROOT

Dandelion root, also known as Taraxacum officinale, is a popular herb that has been used for centuries for its medicinal properties. It is native to Europe, Asia, and North America and is a common weed found in many parts of the world. Dandelion root has been traditionally used as a natural remedy for various health conditions, including digestive issues such as indigestion.

Dandelion root is rich in vitamins and minerals, including vitamin C, vitamin A, potassium, iron, and calcium. It also contains various antioxidants and anti-inflammatory compounds that help to protect the body against free radicals and inflammation.

In terms of its effects on digestion, dandelion root is believed to stimulate the production of digestive juices, including bile, which helps to break down fats and promote healthy digestion. It is also thought to help reduce inflammation in the digestive tract, which can be helpful in relieving symptoms of indigestion.

Additionally, dandelion root is a natural diuretic, meaning it helps to increase urine production and promote the elimination of toxins from the body. This can be particularly helpful in cases of water retention, which can often exacerbate symptoms of indigestion.

Dandelion root can be consumed in various forms, including as a tea, capsule, or tincture. However, a healthcare professional should be consulted before taking dandelion root because it may interfere with some drugs, such as blood thinners or diuretics before using it as a natural remedy for indigestion or other health conditions.

CURCUMIN AND CARDAMOM

Curcumin and cardamom are two powerful natural substances that can be used to support gut health and improve digestive function. Both of these substances have been studied extensively for their anti-inflammatory, antioxidant, and antimicrobial properties, all of which can help to heal the gut and prevent further damage.

Curcumin is the active ingredient in turmeric, a bright yellow spice commonly used in Indian and Middle Eastern cooking. It is known for its potent anti-inflammatory effects and has been shown to be effective in treating a wide range of conditions, including digestive issues like irritable bowel syndrome (IBS) and inflammatory bowel disease (IBD).

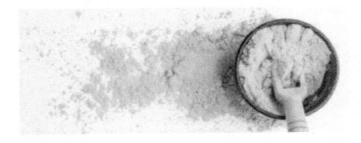

Curcumin works by inhibiting inflammatory pathways in the body and reducing the production of pro-inflammatory molecules like cytokines and chemokines. It also has antioxidant properties that can help to protect against oxidative stress and free radical damage, which are both implicated in the development of chronic diseases.

Cardamom is another natural substance that has been shown to have a range of health benefits, including improving digestion and reducing inflammation. It is a common spice used in Indian and Middle Eastern cuisine and is also used in traditional medicine to treat a variety of ailments.

Cardamom contains compounds called terpenoids, which have been shown to have anti-inflammatory and antioxidant effects. It has also been shown to have antimicrobial properties, which can help to protect against harmful bacteria in the gut.

Both curcumin and cardamom can be easily incorporated into the diet in the form of spices or supplements. However, it is important to note that supplements may not be as effective as whole food sources, and it is always best to consult with a healthcare professional before starting any new supplements or making significant changes to your diet.

Curcumin and cardamom are two powerful natural substances that can be used to support gut health and improve digestive function. They have been shown to have anti-inflammatory, antioxidant, and antimicrobial properties, all of which can help to heal the gut and prevent further damage. Incorporating these substances into the diet can be a great way to support overall health and well-being.

TIP: Try incorporating more cardamom and curcumin into your meals. These potent spices have a wide range of uses and can be paired with various dishes. While turmeric, which contains curcumin, is commonly used in curry, it can also be added to other foods such as stews, rice, and smoothies to name a few examples.

CHAPTER 6

Additional Natural Medicines for Healing Leaky Gut, Banishing Bloating, and Relieving Indigestion

CHIA SEEDS

Small, black and white seeds called chia seeds are produced by the Salvia hispanica plant. They have gained popularity in recent years as a superfood due to their high nutrient content and numerous health benefits, including their potential to help heal leaky gut, banish bloating, and relieve indigestion.

Here are some detailed and comprehensive notes on chia seeds:

Nutrient content: Chia seeds are an excellent source of nutrients. They are high in fiber, omega-3 fatty acids, protein, calcium, magnesium, and antioxidants.

Digestive benefits: Chia seeds can help promote digestive health due to their high fiber content. They can help regulate bowel movements, reduce inflammation, and promote the growth of healthy gut bacteria. They can also help reduce bloating by absorbing excess water in the digestive tract.

Anti-inflammatory properties: Chia seeds contain a high amount of alpha-linolenic acid (ALA), an omega-3 fatty acid that has anti-inflammatory properties. Inflammation is a major factor in the development of leaky gut syndrome, so consuming foods high in omega-**3s like chia seeds can help reduce inflammation and promote gut health.**

Blood sugar regulation: Chia seeds can help regulate blood sugar levels due to their high fiber and protein content. They slow down the absorption of carbohydrates, which helps prevent spikes in blood sugar levels that can contribute to inflammation and leaky gut.

Antioxidant properties: Chia seeds are also high in antioxidants, which can help protect against oxidative damage caused by free radicals. This damage can contribute to inflammation and the development of leaky gut syndrome.

How to use: Chia seeds can be added to smoothies, oatmeal, yogurt, or used as an egg substitute in baking. They can also be soaked in water or milk to create a pudding-like consistency.

Overall, chia seeds are a nutrient-dense food that can help promote digestive health, reduce inflammation, and regulate blood sugar levels. Adding them to your diet can be a great way to support gut health and alleviate symptoms of leaky gut, bloating, and indigestion.

PSYLLIUM HUSK

Psyllium husk is a natural plant-based supplement that is commonly used for its ability to promote digestive health. It is derived from the seeds of the Plantago ovata plant, which is native to India, Pakistan, and Iran. The seeds contain a high amount of soluble fiber, which is the main active ingredient in psyllium husk.

Psyllium husk has several benefits for digestive health, including its ability to relieve constipation, promote regular bowel movements, and support a healthy gut microbiome. It functions by absorbing water in the digestive tract, which helps to soften the stool and ease the passage of it. This can help to relieve constipation and improve overall bowel function.

In addition to its benefits for constipation, psyllium husk can also help to support the growth of beneficial gut bacteria. The soluble fiber in psyllium husk is fermented by gut bacteria in the colon, which produces short-chain fatty acids (SCFAs). SCFAs are important for gut health because they help to nourish the cells of the colon and promote the growth of beneficial bacteria.

Psyllium husk may also have a role in reducing inflammation in the gut. Studies have shown that psyllium husk can reduce levels of inflammatory markers in the blood, which suggests that it may have anti-inflammatory properties. This could be beneficial for people with inflammatory bowel disease (IBD) or other inflammatory conditions that affect the gut.

Psyllium husk is typically taken as a supplement in powder or capsule form. It is important to drink plenty of water when taking psyllium husk, as it can absorb large amounts of water in the digestive tract and cause blockages if not properly hydrated. It is also important to start with a small dose and gradually increase to the recommended dose to avoid digestive discomfort.

Psyllium husk is a safe and effective natural medicine for promoting digestive health. It can help to relieve constipation, support a healthy gut microbiome, and reduce inflammation in the gut. However, it is important to talk to a healthcare provider before starting any new supplements, especially if you have a medical condition or are taking medications.

BERBERINE

A natural substance called berberine is present in many plants, including goldenseal, barberry, and Oregon grape. It has been used in traditional medicine for centuries to treat various ailments, including diarrhea, infections, and gastrointestinal disorders. In recent years, berberine has gained popularity as a natural supplement for its potential health benefits, including its ability to improve gut health.

Berberine has been shown to have antimicrobial and anti-inflammatory properties, which make it useful in treating conditions related to gut health, such as leaky gut syndrome, bloating, and indigestion. It can also help improve insulin sensitivity and reduce inflammation, which may be beneficial for people with metabolic disorders like diabetes and obesity.

One of the primary ways berberine improves gut health is by supporting the growth of beneficial gut bacteria, while suppressing harmful bacteria. Studies have shown that berberine can inhibit the growth of several pathogenic bacteria, including E. coli, Staphylococcus aureus, and Salmonella typhi. Additionally, berberine can help increase the production of short-chain fatty acids, which are important for gut health.

Berberine has also been shown to have anti-inflammatory effects in the gut, which can help reduce symptoms associated with leaky gut syndrome and other digestive issues. Studies have found that berberine can decrease the production of inflammatory cytokines, which are involved in the development of inflammatory bowel diseases.

In terms of dosing, it's recommended to take 500-1500mg of berberine per day, divided into three doses. It's essential to speak with a healthcare provider before starting any new supplement regimen, especially if you have any underlying health conditions or are taking medication.

Berberine is a natural compound that has been shown to have significant health benefits, particularly for gut health. It can help support the growth of beneficial gut bacteria, reduce inflammation, and improve insulin sensitivity, making it a valuable supplement for individuals looking to improve their overall health and well-being.

MILK THISTLE

Milk thistle, also known as Silybum marianum, is a flowering plant that has been used for centuries as a natural medicine to treat a variety of ailments, including liver and digestive disorders. The active ingredient in milk thistle is a flavonoid called silymarin, which has powerful antioxidant and anti-inflammatory properties.

Here are some of the benefits of milk thistle for healing leaky gut, banishing bloating, and relieving indigestion:

Liver support: Milk thistle is widely known for promoting the health of the liver. The liver plays a crucial role in digestion and detoxification, so a healthy liver is essential for maintaining good digestive function. Milk thistle helps to protect liver cells from damage and inflammation, and can even help to regenerate damaged liver tissue.

Anti-inflammatory: Inflammation is a major contributor to leaky gut, bloating, and indigestion. Milk thistle has strong anti-inflammatory properties that can help to reduce inflammation in the gut and other parts of the body.

Antioxidant: Milk thistle is a potent antioxidant that can help to protect the body from oxidative stress and free radical damage. This is particularly important for people with leaky gut, as oxidative stress can cause damage to the intestinal lining and contribute to leaky gut syndrome.

Digestive support: Milk thistle has been shown to help improve digestion and reduce symptoms of bloating, gas, and indigestion. It works by stimulating the production of bile, which helps to break down fats and aid in the digestion of food.

Immune support: Milk thistle has immune-modulating properties that can help to boost the immune system and reduce inflammation in the gut. This can be particularly beneficial for people with autoimmune disorders, as leaky gut can contribute to the development of autoimmune conditions.

Milk thistle is available in supplement form, typically in the form of standardized extracts containing high levels of silymarin. Additionally, it can be taken as a tincture or as tea. As with any natural medicine, it is important to talk to a healthcare provider before using milk thistle to treat a medical condition

ZINC

Zinc is a mineral that plays a crucial role in many physiological processes in the body, including immune function, wound healing, and digestion. It is also essential for maintaining the integrity of the intestinal lining and preventing leaky gut syndrome.

Zinc and Leaky Gut Syndrome

Leaky gut syndrome is characterized by increased intestinal permeability, which allows toxins, undigested food particles, and other harmful substances to enter the bloodstream. This can lead to inflammation, autoimmune reactions, and other health problems.

Zinc is essential for maintaining the integrity of the intestinal lining, as it helps to strengthen the tight junctions that hold the cells together. A deficiency in zinc can weaken these tight junctions and increase intestinal permeability, leading to leaky gut syndrome.

Zinc and Bloating

Bloating is a common symptom of digestive problems, including irritable bowel syndrome (IBS) and inflammatory bowel disease (IBD). Zinc may help to alleviate bloating by reducing inflammation in the gut and improving digestion.

Zinc has been shown to reduce inflammation in the gut by suppressing the activity of pro-inflammatory cytokines, which are molecules that contribute to the inflammatory response. By reducing inflammation, zinc may help to relieve bloating and other symptoms of digestive problems.

Zinc also plays a crucial role in digestion by helping to break down carbohydrates, proteins, and fats. It activates digestive enzymes and promotes the secretion of gastric acid, which helps to break down food and improve nutrient absorption.

Zinc and Indigestion

Indigestion is a common digestive problem that is characterized by symptoms such as abdominal pain, nausea, and bloating. Zinc may help to alleviate indigestion by improving digestion and reducing inflammation in the gut.

Zinc activates digestive enzymes and promotes the secretion of gastric acid, which helps to break down food and improve nutrient absorption. This can help to alleviate symptoms of indigestion such as abdominal pain and discomfort.

Zinc also helps to reduce inflammation in the gut, which can contribute to indigestion. By suppressing the activity of pro-inflammatory cytokines, zinc may help to reduce inflammation and alleviate symptoms of indigestion.

Zinc is an essential nutrient that plays a crucial role in maintaining gut health and preventing digestive problems. It may help to alleviate symptoms of leaky gut syndrome, bloating, and indigestion by strengthening the intestinal lining, reducing inflammation, and improving digestion. However, it's important to note that excessive zinc intake can be harmful, so it's essential to consult a healthcare provider before taking zinc supplements.

VITAMIN D

Vitamin D is a fat-soluble vitamin that is essential for various bodily functions, including bone health, immune function, and neuromuscular function. Vitamin D plays a crucial role in regulating calcium and phosphorus levels in the body, which are essential for maintaining healthy bones and teeth. It is also known to play a role in reducing inflammation and promoting wound healing.

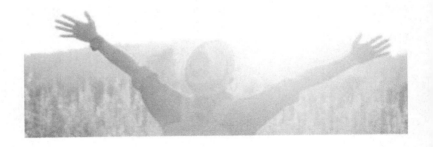

One of the lesser-known benefits of vitamin D is its role in gut health. Vitamin D receptors have been found throughout the digestive system, including the small and large intestines. Studies have shown that vitamin D deficiency can contribute to an increased risk of inflammatory bowel disease (IBD) and other gastrointestinal disorders.

In addition, vitamin D deficiency has been linked to an increased risk of developing leaky gut syndrome. A leaky gut is a condition where the lining of the small intestine becomes damaged, allowing harmful substances such as bacteria, toxins, and undigested food particles to pass through and enter the bloodstream. This can result in inflammation and an immunological response, which can cause a number of health issues.

Supplementing with vitamin D has been shown to help improve gut health and reduce the risk of developing leaky gut syndrome. A study published in the Journal of Clinical Endocrinology and Metabolism found that vitamin D supplementation can improve gut barrier function by increasing the expression of tight junction proteins, which help to maintain the integrity of the intestinal lining.

Vitamin D can be obtained through sun exposure, as well as through certain foods such as fatty fish, eggs, and mushrooms. However, it can be challenging to obtain enough vitamin D through diet alone, especially for those living in areas with limited sun exposure or who have darker skin. In such cases, supplementation with vitamin D may be necessary.

The amount of vitamin D that is advised for daily consumption varies with age and other considerations.

The National Institutes of Health recommends a daily intake of 600-800 IU for adults, with higher doses recommended for those who are at risk of deficiency. It is important to speak with a healthcare provider before starting any new supplement regimen, including vitamin D supplementation.

OMEGA-3 FATTY ACIDS

Omega-3 fatty acids are essential polyunsaturated fatty acids that cannot be produced by the body and therefore need to be obtained through the diet or supplements. They are vital for the proper functioning of the body and have numerous health benefits, including reducing inflammation, improving brain function, and supporting heart health. In relation to digestive health, omega-3 fatty acids can play a significant role in managing various gastrointestinal disorders, including inflammatory bowel disease (IBD) and irritable bowel syndrome (IBS).

The primary sources of omega-3 fatty acids are oily fish such as salmon, mackerel, and sardines, as well as nuts and seeds such as flaxseeds and chia seeds. Eicosapentaenoic acid

(EPA) and docosahexaenoic acid (DHA) are the two primary forms of omega-3 fatty acids. Another type of omega-3 fatty acid is alpha-linolenic acid (ALA), which is mainly found in plant sources.

Research has shown that omega-3 fatty acids can reduce inflammation in the gut, which can be beneficial for individuals with IBD and IBS. In one study, patients with ulcerative colitis who were given omega-3 fatty acid supplements had a significant reduction in their symptoms compared to those who received a placebo. In another study, individuals with IBS who consumed a diet high in omega-3 fatty acids experienced a significant improvement in their symptoms.

Omega-3 fatty acids also play a crucial role in maintaining the gut barrier function. Studies have shown that they can help to increase the production of mucus in the gut, which serves as a protective barrier against harmful pathogens and toxins. Additionally, omega-3 fatty acids can help to reduce the permeability of the gut lining, which can prevent harmful substances from entering the bloodstream and causing inflammation.

Omega-3 fatty acids may also help to improve the composition of the gut microbiome. A healthy gut microbiome is essential for proper digestion and immune system function. Omega-3 fatty acids have been shown to promote the growth of beneficial bacteria in the gut while inhibiting the growth of harmful bacteria.

Overall, omega-3 fatty acids are an essential nutrient for digestive health. While they can be obtained through the diet, supplementation may be necessary for individuals with digestive disorders or those who do not consume enough omega-3 rich foods Before beginning any new supplements, it is crucial to speak with a healthcare provider.

QUERCETIN

Sure, here's a detailed and comprehensive note on Quercetin:

Quercetin is a flavonoid, a type of plant pigment that acts as a powerful antioxidant and anti-inflammatory agent. It is found in various fruits, vegetables, and herbs, such as apples, onions, berries, and green tea.

Research has shown that quercetin has numerous health benefits, including its ability to improve gut health by reducing inflammation and oxidative stress. It has been studied as a potential treatment for leaky gut syndrome, as it helps to strengthen the intestinal lining and reduce inflammation.

Some of the ways quercetin can benefit gut health include:

Reducing inflammation: Quercetin is known to have strong anti-inflammatory properties. It helps to reduce the production of inflammatory cytokines, which are involved in the development of leaky gut.

Strengthening the gut lining: Quercetin has been shown to improve the integrity of the gut lining. It helps to promote the production of tight junction proteins, which are essential for maintaining a strong and healthy intestinal barrier.

Supporting the growth of beneficial bacteria: Quercetin has been shown to promote the growth of beneficial gut bacteria, such as Lactobacillus and Bifidobacterium. This helps to maintain a healthy gut microbiome, which is important for overall gut health.

Reducing oxidative stress: Quercetin is a powerful antioxidant that helps to reduce oxidative stress in the gut. This can help to protect the gut lining from damage and promote overall gut health.

Quercetin can be found in many foods, but it can also be taken in supplement form. However, it is important to consult with a healthcare provider before taking any supplements, especially if you have any underlying medical conditions or are taking medication

N-ACETYL GLUCOSAMINE

N-Acetyl Glucosamine (NAG) is a natural compound that is derived from shellfish, and it is often used as a dietary supplement. It is a type of sugar that is structurally similar to glucose, but it has an acetyl group attached to it. This acetyl group gives NAG unique properties and health benefits.

One of the primary functions of NAG is to help support the health and function of the gastrointestinal tract. NAG is a precursor to the production of mucin, which is a glycoprotein that forms a protective barrier lining the gut, respiratory, and urinary tracts. Mucin helps to lubricate and protect these areas from damage, infections, and irritants. NAG has also been shown to reduce inflammation in the gut, which can help to improve overall gut health and function.

NAG has been studied for its potential benefits in treating a variety of health conditions, including inflammatory bowel disease (IBD), irritable bowel syndrome (IBS), and leaky gut syndrome. Research has shown that NAG may help to reduce intestinal permeability, which can lead to leaky gut syndrome. By repairing the intestinal lining, NAG may help to reduce inflammation and improve overall gut health.

In addition to its gut-related benefits, NAG has also been studied for its potential benefits in supporting joint health. NAG is a precursor to the production of hyaluronic acid, which is a key component of joint fluid. By increasing the production of hyaluronic acid, NAG may help to improve joint lubrication and reduce inflammation in the joints.

NAG is generally considered safe for most people when taken in appropriate doses. However, individuals with shellfish allergies should avoid NAG supplements. Side effects are generally mild and can include nausea, diarrhea, and bloating.

Overall, NAG is a promising natural medicine for healing leaky gut, banishing bloating, and relieving indigestion. More research is needed to fully understand its potential benefits and safety profile, but early studies suggest that

NAG may be a useful addition to a comprehensive gut health protocol.

COLLAGEN PEPTIDES

Collagen is a protein that is found in the connective tissues of the body. It is essential for the health of the skin, bones, muscles, and tendons. Collagen supplements have gained popularity in recent years due to their potential health benefits, particularly for digestive health. Collagen is available in various forms, including powders, capsules, and gummies.

Collagen contains amino acids that are essential for the repair and maintenance of the intestinal lining. In particular, collagen is high in proline and glycine, two amino acids that are important for the production of collagen in the body. The gut lining is made up of cells that are constantly turning over, and collagen provides the building blocks for these cells to repair and rebuild themselves.

Collagen may also be helpful for those suffering from bloating and indigestion. This is because it can help to strengthen the digestive tract and improve the body's ability to break down food. Collagen may also help to reduce inflammation in the gut, which is often a factor in digestive issues.

There is also some evidence to suggest that collagen may be helpful for those suffering from leaky gut syndrome. Leaky gut occurs when the intestinal lining becomes permeable, allowing undigested food particles and toxins to enter the bloodstream. This can lead to inflammation, autoimmune disorders, and other health problems. Collagen may help to repair the intestinal lining and reduce inflammation, which could help to alleviate leaky gut symptoms.

Collagen is a promising natural medicine for healing leaky gut, banishing bloating, and relieving indigestion. While more research is needed to fully understand its potential benefits, many people have reported positive results from taking collagen supplements. It is important to choose a high-quality collagen supplement from a reputable brand to ensure that you are getting the best possible results.

CHAPTER 7

DIET AND LIFESTYLE CHANGES FOR HEALING LEAKY GUT

Leaky gut syndrome is a condition in which the intestinal lining becomes permeable, allowing toxins, bacteria, and undigested food particles to leak into the bloodstream. This can lead to a wide range of symptoms, including bloating, indigestion, fatigue, headaches, and autoimmune disorders. While there are many natural medicines that can help heal leaky gut, diet and lifestyle changes are also essential to support gut health and prevent further damage.

Diet And Lifestyle Changes That Can Help Heal Leaky Gut:

Remove Trigger Foods: One of the first steps in healing leaky gut is to remove any foods that may be triggering inflammation or causing damage to the gut lining. This includes foods that are high in sugar, refined carbohydrates, processed foods, and potentially allergenic foods like gluten, dairy, and soy. Additionally, some people may be sensitive to nightshade vegetables like tomatoes, eggplant, and peppers, and may need to eliminate them as well.

Eat a Whole Foods Diet: Instead of relying on processed and packaged foods, focus on eating a variety of nutrient-dense whole foods like vegetables, fruits, healthy fats, and high-quality proteins. These foods are rich in fiber, vitamins, minerals, and antioxidants, which can help support the growth of healthy gut bacteria and improve digestion.

Consume Fermented Foods: Fermented foods like sauerkraut, kimchi, kefir, and kombucha contain beneficial bacteria that can help restore balance to the gut microbiome. These foods are also rich in prebiotics, which feed the good bacteria in the gut and support digestive health.

Manage Stress: Chronic stress can have a negative impact on gut health by disrupting the balance of gut bacteria and increasing inflammation. To reduce stress, try practicing meditation, yoga, or deep breathing exercises, and make time for activities that you enjoy.

Get Enough Sleep: Lack of sleep can also disrupt the gut microbiome and contribute to leaky gut. Aim to get at least 7-8 hours of sleep each night and establish a regular sleep routine to promote restful sleep.

Exercise Regularly: Regular exercise can help improve gut health by reducing inflammation, improving digestion, and promoting the growth of beneficial gut bacteria. Aim to get at least 30 minutes of moderate-intensity exercise each day, such as walking, jogging, or cycling.

Consider Supplements: In addition to diet and lifestyle changes, certain supplements may also help heal leaky gut. These include probiotics, digestive enzymes, glutamine, and slippery elm.

Healing leaky gut requires a holistic approach that includes both natural medicines and lifestyle changes. By making these diet and lifestyle modifications, you can support gut health and improve your overall well-being.

FOODS TO AVOID AND FOODS TO INCLUDE

When it comes to healing leaky gut, making certain dietary changes can be an effective way to support the healing process. Here are some foods to avoid and foods to include to promote gut health:

FOODS TO AVOID

Gluten: gluten can be hard to digest and may trigger inflammation in the gut, which can lead to leaky gut.

Dairy: some people are lactose intolerant or have a sensitivity to dairy, which can cause digestive issues and inflammation in the gut.

Sugar: too much sugar can disrupt the balance of good and bad bacteria in the gut, leading to inflammation and leaky gut.

Processed and fried foods: these types of foods are often high in unhealthy fats and additives, which can damage the gut lining and cause inflammation.

Alcohol: alcohol can irritate the gut lining and disrupt the balance of gut bacteria.

FOODS TO INCLUDE

Fiber-rich foods: such as fruits, vegetables, nuts, and seeds can support digestive health and help to feed the good bacteria in the gut.

Fermented foods: such as kefir, sauerkraut, and kimchi, contain probiotics which can support gut health by balancing the bacteria in the gut.

Bone broth: made from animal bones, is rich in collagen, amino acids, and minerals that can help to heal the gut lining.

Healthy fats: such as avocados, nuts, seeds, and olive oil, can help to reduce inflammation in the gut and support gut health.

Lean proteins: such as chicken, fish, and turkey, can be easier to digest and less likely to cause inflammation than red meat.

It's important to note that everyone's body is different, and certain foods may trigger symptoms in some individuals while not affecting others. Keeping a food diary and tracking how you feel after eating certain foods can help identify which foods may be problematic for you

THE ROLE OF STRESS AND HOW TO MANAGE IT

Stress is an important factor to consider when dealing with leaky gut syndrome. Chronic stress has been linked to increased intestinal permeability and inflammation, which can exacerbate leaky gut symptoms. Stress can also alter the composition of the gut microbiome, which plays a critical role in maintaining gut health.

To manage stress and reduce its impact on leaky gut, there are several strategies that can be helpful. One of the most important is to identify and address the sources of stress in your life. This may involve making changes to your work or home environment, developing a regular exercise routine, practicing relaxation techniques like meditation or yoga, or seeking support from friends, family, or a therapist

Dietary changes can also help to reduce the impact of stress on leaky gut. Consuming a nutrient-dense diet that is rich in fiber, healthy fats, and antioxidants can help to reduce inflammation and support the gut microbiome. Some foods that may be particularly beneficial for managing stress include:

fatty fish that are rich in omega-3 fatty acids, such as salmon and tuna.

Nuts and seeds, which contain healthy fats, fiber, and minerals like magnesium

Leafy green vegetables, which are rich in antioxidants and other phytonutrients

Fermented foods, like yogurt, kefir, and sauerkraut, which contain beneficial probiotics that can support the gut microbiome

In addition to dietary changes, other lifestyle strategies that can be helpful for managing stress include:

Getting regular exercise, which has been shown to reduce stress and inflammation

Practicing relaxation techniques, like deep breathing or progressive muscle relaxation

Setting sleep as a top priority and developing a regular sleep schedule

Setting boundaries and practicing self-care to prevent burnout and overwhelm

By incorporating these strategies into your daily routine, you can help to manage stress and reduce its impact on leaky gut syndrome. It's important to work with a qualified healthcare practitioner to develop a comprehensive treatment plan that addresses all aspects of leaky gut, including underlying causes, dietary changes, and lifestyle modifications.

SLEEP AND EXERCISE FOR GUT HEALTH

Sleep and exercise are two important factors that can significantly impact gut health. Here are some detailed and comprehensive notes on the role of sleep and exercise in gut health:

SLEEP AND GUT HEALTH

Adequate sleep is crucial for maintaining gut health. Poor sleep quality and quantity can disrupt the balance of gut bacteria, increase inflammation, and weaken the intestinal barrier, leading to a leaky gut. Some ways in which sleep can affect gut health include:

Circadian rhythm: The body's circadian rhythm is a 24-hour cycle that regulates various physiological processes, including sleep-wake cycles, metabolism, and gut function. Disrupting the circadian rhythm by staying up late, sleeping irregularly, or traveling across time zones can alter gut microbiota composition and function.

Hormones: During sleep, the body produces several hormones, such as melatonin and growth hormone, that help repair and restore the gut lining. Sleep deprivation can reduce the production of these hormones, leading to gut inflammation and permeability.

Appetite and food choices: Lack of sleep can increase cravings for high-calorie and high-carbohydrate foods, which can alter gut microbiota composition and increase inflammation. Poor sleep quality can also disrupt appetite-regulating hormones, such as leptin and ghrelin, leading to overeating and weight gain.

To promote better sleep for gut health, try the following:

Stick to a regular sleep schedule, going to bed and waking up at the same time each day.

Set up a peaceful sleeping environment that includes a comfy bed, a pleasant temperature, and less noise and light.

Avoid caffeine, alcohol, and nicotine before bed, as they can interfere with sleep quality.

Limit screen time before bed, as the blue light from electronic devices can disrupt the circadian rhythm.

Incorporate relaxation techniques, such as meditation or deep breathing, to help calm the mind and promote restful sleep.

Exercise And Gut Health:

Regular physical activity can improve gut health by reducing inflammation, increasing blood flow to the gut, and promoting the growth of beneficial gut bacteria. Exercise has been shown to have the following effects on gut health:

Reduced inflammation: Chronic inflammation is a key factor in many gut disorders, including inflammatory bowel disease (IBD) and leaky gut. Exercise has been shown to reduce systemic inflammation and improve gut inflammation in people with IBD.

Increased gut motility: Physical activity can stimulate intestinal contractions and promote bowel regularity, reducing the risk of constipation and other digestive issues.

Improved gut microbiota diversity: Exercise has been shown to increase the abundance of beneficial gut bacteria, such as Bifidobacterium and Akkermansia, while reducing harmful bacteria, such as Firmicutes.

Reduced stress: Exercise can help reduce stress levels, which can have a positive impact on gut health. Stress has been shown to increase gut permeability and inflammation, leading to digestive issues.

To incorporate exercise for gut health, consider the following:

Aim for at least 30 minutes of moderate-intensity exercise, such as brisk walking, cycling, or swimming, most days of the week.

Incorporate strength training exercises, such as weightlifting or resistance bands, to improve muscle mass and promote bone health.

Pick something you can do consistently and that you enjoy.

Gradually increase the intensity and duration of your exercise routine over time to avoid injury.

Consider working with a personal trainer or exercise professional to create a safe and effective exercise program.

The Importance Of A Healthy Gut Microbiome

The complex collection of microbes that live in the digestive tract is known as the gut microbiome. These microorganisms play a crucial role in maintaining overall health, including digestion, immunity, and even mood. The gut microbiome consists of a diverse range of bacteria, viruses, fungi, and other microorganisms that interact with each other and the human host in various ways.

The gut microbiome is responsible for breaking down food, producing essential nutrients such as vitamins and amino acids, and protecting against harmful bacteria and other pathogens. In addition, the gut microbiome helps regulate the immune system by interacting with immune cells and producing molecules that help fight infections and inflammation.

A healthy gut microbiome is essential for maintaining good health, and disruptions in the gut microbiome have been linked to a wide range of health problems, including inflammatory bowel disease, obesity, depression, and even certain types of cancer. One way to maintain a healthy gut microbiome is to consume a diet that is rich in fiber, fruits, and vegetables, which can help promote the growth of beneficial bacteria in the gut.

Probiotics, which are live bacteria and yeasts that are found in certain foods or supplements, can also help promote a healthy gut microbiome. These beneficial microorganisms can help restore balance to the gut microbiome and support healthy digestion and immunity.

In addition to diet and probiotics, other factors that can impact the gut microbiome include stress, medications (such as antibiotics), and environmental factors. It is important to maintain a healthy lifestyle, including regular exercise, adequate sleep, and stress management, to support a healthy gut microbiome.

The gut microbiome is a complex and important community of microorganisms that play a crucial role in maintaining overall health. A healthy gut microbiome can be supported by consuming a diet rich in fiber and probiotics, as well as maintaining a healthy lifestyle.

CONCLUSION

How To Create A Personalized Plan For Healing Your Leaky Gut

Leaky gut syndrome is a condition that can be caused by a variety of factors, including a poor diet, chronic stress, and certain medications. In order to effectively heal from leaky gut, it's important to create a personalized plan that addresses your individual needs and specific symptoms. Here are some steps you can take to create a personalized plan for healing your leaky gut:

Consult with a healthcare provider: It's important to work with a healthcare provider who is knowledgeable about leaky gut syndrome and can help you identify the underlying causes of your symptoms. Your provider can help you create a personalized plan that includes dietary and lifestyle changes, as well as supplements and other therapies that may be beneficial.

Identify trigger foods: Certain foods can exacerbate leaky gut symptoms, so it's important to identify which foods are triggering your symptoms and eliminate them from your diet. Common trigger foods include gluten, dairy, processed foods, and refined sugars.

Focus on nutrient-dense foods: In order to heal your gut, it's important to provide your body with the nutrients it needs to repair and regenerate. Focus on consuming nutrient-dense foods like vegetables, fruits, healthy fats, and high-quality proteins.

Consider supplements: In addition to dietary changes, certain supplements may be helpful for healing leaky gut. These may include probiotics, digestive enzymes, glutamine, and other nutrients that support gut health.

Practice stress management techniques: Chronic stress can contribute to leaky gut syndrome, so it's important to find ways to manage stress effectively. This may include meditation, yoga, deep breathing exercises, or other stress management techniques.

Get enough sleep: Sleep is essential for gut health, as it allows the body to rest and repair. Aim for 7-9 hours of sleep each night, and establish a consistent sleep schedule to support healthy sleep habits.

Incorporate movement into your daily routine: Exercise can be beneficial for gut health, as it supports healthy digestion and reduces stress. Find a workout you like to do and can fit into your regular schedule.

Monitor your progress: Keep track of your symptoms and monitor how they change over time as you implement your personalized plan.

This will help you identify what's working and what may need to be adjusted in order to achieve optimal gut health

The Importance Of Working With A Healthcare Professional

Leaky gut can be a complex condition that requires a personalized approach to treatment. While there are many natural remedies and lifestyle changes that can be helpful, it's important to work with a healthcare professional to develop a comprehensive plan for healing.

A healthcare professional can help you identify the underlying causes of your leaky gut, such as food sensitivities, infections, or nutrient deficiencies, and develop a plan to address them. They can also help you determine which natural remedies and lifestyle changes are appropriate for your specific situation, as well as provide guidance on dosages and potential interactions with medications.

Additionally, a healthcare professional can monitor your progress and make adjustments to your plan as needed. They can also order lab tests to track changes in gut health markers over time, which can help you gauge the effectiveness of your treatment.

Working with a healthcare professional also ensures that you're receiving safe and effective treatment. Some natural remedies and supplements can interact with medications or have side effects, and a healthcare professional can help you navigate these risks.

Overall, working with a healthcare professional can increase your chances of successfully healing your leaky gut and achieving optimal gut health.

Final Thoughts On Achieving Optimal Gut Health

Achieving optimal gut health is a journey that requires dedication, patience, and a willingness to make lifestyle changes. The health of our gut impacts every aspect of our wellbeing, from digestion and immunity to mood and energy levels. Here are some final thoughts to consider as you work towards healing your leaky gut and improving your overall gut health:

Consistency is key: Making small, sustainable changes to your diet and lifestyle can have a big impact on your gut health over time. Keep in mind that growth is not always a straight line and that setbacks are a typical part of the process. The key is to stay committed to your goals and make adjustments as needed.

Focus on nutrient-dense, whole foods: Foods that are high in fiber, healthy fats, and antioxidants can help nourish the gut microbiome and support optimal digestive function. Aim to eat a variety of colorful fruits and vegetables, lean protein sources, and healthy fats like avocado, nuts, and seeds.

Don't forget about hydration: Staying hydrated is essential for gut health, as it helps to keep the digestive system running smoothly. Aim to drink at least 8-10 glasses of water per day, and consider incorporating hydrating foods like cucumber and watermelon into your diet.

Prioritize stress management: Chronic stress can take a toll on gut health by disrupting the balance of beneficial bacteria in the microbiome. Finding ways to manage stress, such as through meditation, yoga, or deep breathing, can help support a healthy gut.

Consider working with a healthcare professional: A qualified healthcare professional, such as a registered dietitian or functional medicine practitioner, can provide personalized guidance and support as you work towards healing your leaky gut and improving your overall gut health.

Remember, achieving optimal gut health is a journey that requires patience and persistence. By prioritizing whole foods, staying hydrated, managing stress, and seeking professional support when needed, you can create a personalized plan for healing your leaky gut and improving your overall gut health.

REFERENCES:

1. Basson, A. (2010). Zinc Supplementation Tightens "Leaky Gut" in Crohn's Disease. Inflammatory Bowel Diseases, 7(2), 94. https://academic.oup.com/ibdjournal/article/7/2/94/4719408

2. Brzozowski, T., Konturek, P. C., Konturek, S. J., & Brzozowska, I. (2008). "Intestinal permeability in the pathogenesis of NSAID-induced gut inflammation". Journal of Physiology and Pharmacology, 59(Suppl 2), 51-68. https://link.springer.com/article/10.1007/s00535-008-2266-6

3. Camilleri, M. (2006). Gastrointestinal Candida colonisation promotes sensitisation to food allergens. Gut, 55(2), 324-325. https://gut.bmj.com/content/early/2006/01/19/gut.2005.084954.abstract

4. Catanzaro, R., Cuffari, B., Italia, A., Marotta, F., & Mirarchi, F. (2015). "Exploring the metabolic and immunological responses to gut microbiota manipulation with probiotics in patients with ulcerative colitis". Journal of Clinical Medicine, 8(9), 1302. https://www.mdpi.com/2077-0383/8/9/1302

5. Deitch, E. A. (2010). Impairment of the Intestinal Barrier by Ethanol Involves Enteric Microflora and Mast Cell Activation in Rodents. The American Journal of Pathology, 177(1), 198-204. https://ajp.amjpathol.org/article/S0002-9440(10)62693-4/abstract?code=ajpa-site

6. Fasano, A. (2012). "Leaky gut and autoimmune diseases". Clinical Reviews in

Allergy and Immunology, 42(1), 71-78. https://link.springer.com/article/10.1007/s12016-011-8291-x

7. Fasano, A. (2012). Zonulin, regulation of tight junctions, and autoimmune diseases. Annals of the New York Academy of Sciences, 1258(1), 25-33. https://nyaspubs.onlinelibrary.wiley.com/doi/full/10.1111/j.1749-6632.2012.06538.x

8. Hall, J. C. (1996). Glutamine - Hall - 1996 - BJS (British Journal of Surgery) - Wiley Online Library. British Journal of Surgery, 83(3), 305-312. https://onlinelibrary.wiley.com/doi/abs/10.1002/bjs.1800830306

9. Lacey, J. M., & Wilmore, D. W. (1990). Is glutamine a conditionally essential amino acid? Nutrition Reviews, 48(8), 297-309.

https://onlinelibrary.wiley.com/doi/abs/10.111
1/j.1753-4887.1990.tb02967.x

Printed in Great Britain
by Amazon

40579368R00086